GOUT AND ITS CURE

BY

J. COMPTON BURNETT, M. D.

"Das, was die Exkremente macht, was die *Fœces* im Leibe macht, die Du *Humores* heissest, dieselbe sind nicht die Krankheit. Das ist die Krankheit, die dasselbe macht, dass es also wird. Wer seihet dasselbe? Niemand. Wer greift es? Niemand. Wie kann denn ein Arzt *in humoribus* die Krankheit suchen und ihren Ursprung melden aus denselben, dieweil sie von der Krankheit werden geboren, und nicht die Krankheit von ihnen?"—HOHENHEIM.

B. JAIN PUBLISHERS (P) Ltd.
DELHI

Price : Rs. 25.00

Reprint Edition 2001

© Copyright with Publishers

Published by:
B. Jain Publishers (P) Ltd.
1921, Street No. 10th Chuna Mandi,
Paharganj, New Delhi-110055 (INDIA)

Printed in India by:
Unisons Techno Financial Consultants (P) Ltd.
522, FIE, Patpar Ganj, Delhi- 110 092.

ISBN 81-7021-634-6
BOOK CODE B-2128

PREFACE.

For the successful treatment of gout it is
necessary to have a clear idea of what
constitutes its various parts ; notably must
we differentiate between its pre-deposit
symptoms and its post-deposit symptoms,
for much of the want of success in its cure
is due to a mixing-up of the two sets of
symptoms. The symptoms that precede
and lead up to the uric acid retentions in
the blood are a series by themselves ; those
due to the uric acid in the blood and which
lead up to the gouty deposit as an attack,
or as chronic deposits, are a second series.
The former really spell arthritic cacopepsia,
while the latter are synonymous with uric
acid poisoning ; in the one we deal with the
producing power, in the other with the
product.

This differentiation being made, we proceed on two lines with the treatment,—the one to get rid of the gouty attack and the deposits, and the other, the more important, to deal with that which leads to the production of the uric material.

The following pages are intended to set forth the writer's method of procedure.

J. COMPTON BURNETT.

86 WIMPOLE STREET, W.,
January, 1895.

Gout and its Cure.

GOUT AND ITS CURE.

THE various conditions known
or thought to be manifestations of gout lie on either side of
every medical path, and most
medical practitioners have to deal
with them in some form or another.
Gout in this country is so common,
that not a few persons are in the
habit of treating their gouty attacks
with their family doctor's favorite
preparation of *Colchicum*, aided, or
supposedly aided, by a liver-pill
and alkalies, such as lithia, potash,
or soda. Most of us have our own

notions of the right diet for the
gouty; and as to drinkables, a smart
lady in the North once remarked
to me (on hearing me tell my
patient to drink Scotch whisky
well diluted with water), "Oh ! I
see you are a *Scotch*-whisky doctor.
It seems to me that the only
difference between you gout doctors
lies in the kind of whisky you
order ; you order Scotch, and
Dr. Moore used to order Irish. I
often tell papa that if I were he I
would drink both, and then he
would be sure to be right." The
sting of the remark lay in the fact
that I had the local reputation of
being strongly opposed to alcohol
in any and every form, notably in
the treatment of gout, and the
partial modification of my views

came about in this wise :—I was
once attending a country squire for
an inflamed knee, when his aged
father-in-law, the late Sir Edward
X., then over 80 years of age, came
over to see him. While there on a
visit, he had a smart attack of gout,
which I was called upon to treat,
but my *Aconite* and *Bryonia* did not
help either him or me. *Colchicum*
I would not give, and, moreover, I
did not allow him any alcohol at
all. I had been taught that alcohol
made gout, and so I felt it to
be my duty to get rid of the
cause first, and then the feverishness was met by the *Aconite*,
and the pains and swelling by
Bryonia (pains worse from move-
ment). All that seemed simple
enough ; only Sir Edward got

worse, and told me very plainly
that he did not believe in my new-
fangled treatment of gout at all,
exclaiming, "My little doctor always gets me round in a week or
ten days." Said little doctor was
telegraphed for, and sure enough
he had Sir Edward out driving in
the park in about a week.

What was the little doctor's
treatment? Port wine!

Said he to me: "You see, Sir
Edward's not really a strong man
and never was, although he has
held on a pretty big span; still he
is really a weak man, and he never
could stand anything unless you
stoked him up a bit."

How long has Sir Edward been
your patient

"Forty years."

Have you always "stoked him up" as you say?

"Oh yes, always."

Why?

"Because I found I never could get him well of anything without plenty of port wine."

Do you treat many cases of gout?

"Oh no, very few; people in my district are too poor to get the gout; they work too hard. I get it occasionally myself."

Do you take plenty of port wine yourself?

"No, no; it would kill me."

But you cure Sir Edward with port wine and yourself not; what do you take yourself?

"Oranges, if they are to be got."
Oranges ?

"Yes, I eat two oranges three or four times a day ; drink plenty of clean cold water ; avoid game and beef ; live on plenty of green stuff, particularly salads ; keep my skin clean and active, and I soon get rid of the enemy."

And what about alcohol ? are you a teetotaler ?

"No, not a bit of it, *except when I am gouty;* then I go on oranges and plenty of cold water, and I soon wash out the gout, and then I go on as usual and take whatever is going ; with my big country practice, long distances, and small fees, I cannot be bothered with diet ; bread and cheese, beer, and bread and milk, bacon and eggs, or bread and butter and eggs, are what I usually get at my patients' homes."

The little doctor could give me no guiding rule as to the best diet in gout, viz., when to give plenty of port wine, or when to rely upon oranges and plenty of water. But from subsequent observation I have been able to arrive at the following conclusions, viz. :—

1. People who have descended from ancestors long accustomed to the use of stimulants generation after generation, these need stimulants in their debilitating illness, and therefore in their attacks of gout. They also need a certain amount of building up. If they are dieted too severely and deprived

of their alcoholic stimulants they get weaker and weaker, and their gout gets the entire mastery; whereas with a sustaining diet and a reasonable amount of stimulant, they get well and thrive on their ancestral constitutional basis.

2. In certain brain-workers (and in their immediate descendants) whose nervous systems are exhausted, if you take away their stimulants they are apt to fare very badly.

3. This exhaustion gout, when produced by abstemiousness, can be cured by better diet and stimulants. I knew (socially, not professionally) an eminent Q.C. who had been for many years a total abstainer, lived very sparingly, but who was a

martyr to chronic gout, and eventually died of it about 60 years of age. He was a great brain-worker, and of strong constitution. He was often asked to take some stimulants, but strenuously refused.

4. A gouty patient, who afterwards came under my care, was dieted by a famous anti-fat doctor, and in a week or two he developed a terrible attack of gout that completely broke his seemingly powerful constitution. During the fasting experiments of certain persons at the Royal Aquarium here in London, frequently done during the past few years, the fasters had, over and over again, attacks of gout, though water only was partaken of.

So I conclude that food and

stimulants *per se* are not necessarily the cause of gouty attacks. The things presents itself to my mind thus :—Just as in the case of a smoky chimney almost any kind of fuel will fill the room with smoke, so in gout almost any kind of food will produce gout ; but the real fault lies, not in the fuel, but in the chimney ; not in the food, but in the organism.

I call these cases of gout *Exhaustion Gout*, and certainly they need stimulants.

I have reason to believe that Sir James Paget holds a view something like this, though he may possibly express it differently ; for I once ordered a gentleman who consulted me for what I considered exhaustion gout, to take two glasses of sound port daily with his dessert after dinner, but he refused compliance, and walked out of my consulting-room straight over to see Sir James Paget, telling Sir James nought of having been to see me. Oddly enough Sir James also ordered him a stimulant (though I forget what), and on his objecting to take any stimulant on the ground that it would increase his gout, Sir James said, "Never mind your gout ; get up your strength, and then you will be better able to master your gout." Clearly in these cases of exhaustion gout we have to do with a very different affair to that which yields to oranges and cold water.

Surfeit Gout.

I call surfeit gout that which is
Curable by abstemiousness either as
regards food or stimulants, or both.
In such cases I have known an
attack of gout to be brought on by
a single bottle of beer or a pint of
even the driest champagne, and
on one occasion from eating gooseberries ; in such cases all alcoholic
stimulants, and certain foods, yet
in different degrees, act like oil on
a fire ; they set up a blaze.

In exhaustion gout alcoholic
stimulants act like oil on troubled
waters : they calm the waves.

Exhaustion Gout And Surfeit Gout In The Same Individual.

There are, further, cases of gout that seem to partake of both qualities—*exhaustion* and *surfeit*—and here the question of stimulants is very difficult to decide; on the whole, I have obtained my best curative results by changing the kind of stimulant instead of allowing them to stick to one kind. Thus I have rather a *penchant* for allowing a small quantity of dry champagne for dinner once or twice a week, the same quantity of a sound claret once or twice a week, and whisky and water, or whisky and soda-water, on other days. Allowance must always be made for hereditary proclivities, habits and modes of life. We must ever keep before our minds that in the treatment of gout we are dealing with adults and not with children ; our concern is not to dictate an ideal dietary for the normal individual under hypothetically perfect conditions, but we have to do with sufferers from gout, whom it is our business to get well, and keep well and vigorous as long as possible. In other words, rearing children requires a very different regimen and pietary to what experience may find best for maintaining gouty adults.

Neither is it desirable to limit a gouty man or woman to the barest necessaries of life, and say, it is possible to live on bread, fruit, and clean water, therefore you must eat

nought but bread and fruit, and
drink only the ale that Adam drank.

Taken in its simple elementary
forms, we may regard the exhaustion gout and the surfeit gout as
respectively inherited or acquired.
In the most simple form the heredi-
tarily gouty may get gout on almost any diet. Surfeit gout is self-
produced by exessive input or inadequate output; too much is put
in, too little is put out, and hence
the *ureal smoke and soot* which is
the gouty product. A gouty father
begets a child while he is actively
gouty; like begets like, and hence
the offspring is of necessity gouty
on any diet whatsoever; such
children pass grit and gravel as
soon as they get away from the
pure milk diet. A milk cure for

gout echoes all down through time. But active, middle-aged men in the full swing of daily life com monly find a milk diet inadequate if they keep at work "It does not seem to satisfy me," say they ; or "even when I am full of milk I seem to be empty." The fact is, milk is food for the very young— calves and babes.

Goutiness.

Gout is an acute disease, and shows itself paroxysmally, though the word also expresses the con- stitutional crasis or state ; and so frequently is this latter the case, that I have time and again heard patients exclaim, "Oh ! everything is gout with the doctors now !"

When we say "gout" we really mean that the individual lives goutily, whether such individual gets attacks of gout or not ; thus the child of a gouty father may teethe goutily and have gouty urticaria, and here the gouty quality cannot be eliminated by gumlancing or soothing ointments.

Assuming that both parents of a given individual are pronouncedly gouty, how should the offspring be other than gouty ? In the painful menstruation of young ladies I have over and over again cured the dysmenorrhoea by treating the painful affection as of gouty quality,— in fact, as gout. It would be better to restrict the term gout to the form of disease that occurs in attacks of paroxysmal arthritis, and use the

word goutiness to designate the
more or less hereditary quality of
the constitutional crasis. In fact.
I would use the words goutiness
and gout to indicate the same relation which consumptiveness bears
to consumption. But in this matter of terminology custom will fix
our words for us, no matter what
we say or do.

What Is Gout ?

It would take more time than I
have to spare to enter upon the
subject of what gout really is, by
going over the innumerable theories
that have been advanced from the
year one until now. One line of
thought, however, runs right
through most of them, viz., some
reference is made to the urine or to

one or other of its constituents, according to the terminology current at the time, such as tartarus, stone, gravel, grit, urea, uric acid, urate of sodium. The names of the disease have very little interest, because gout in its ordinary paroxysmal manifestation, *quoad* its *habitat*, will always be a podagra, a cheir-agra, which says but little. Deriving gout from *gutta* via *goutte* is etymologically not without interest, but clinically of no value, whereas the names that refer to its uric or urinous nature do roughly indicate the nature of its product. My own notion of the nature of gout may be expressed in a very few words : *The gouty product is the uric smoke and soot of the human economy,*—that is, the pure paroxysmal affection

commonly manifesting itself as podagra, and more or less in many
varities of goutiness.

The thing presents itself to my
mind thus :—Given the human organism, it takes up its food, use it,
and then gets rid of the products of
its vital phenomena, first by way of
the bowels and then by way of the
skin and kidneys. Where the renal
excretion is such that some of the
uric matter (urea, uric acid, urate
of sodium) remains in the blood, it
is deposited in certain of the tissues, and when it culminates in,
say, the big toe, we get the classic
gouty attack. I am for the moment
not concerned with the precise form
of the urea as so deposited, nor yet
whether due to one cause or another, but with the simple elemen-

tary conception of the substantive
material nature of the gouty product.—in other words, gout, for me,
is ureal poisoning. Of course I part
company with all those who regard
gout as merely uric acid deposits,
and who maintain that the uric
acid is the disease. I grant that the
uric acid produces the sufferings,
but I maintain that the *disease gout*
is that which produces the uric acid,
—in fact, the Paracelsic motto on
my title-page expresses exactly my
philosophy. Pretty well all the
phenomena of gout square well
with this conception of its nature.
It seems to me, further, that gout
stands in some relation to the spleen
as well as to the kidneys and sweat
glands. It does not appear to me
that gout has so much to do with

the liver or its functions, and stirring up the liver to increased action and purging the bowels do not, so far as I have been able to discover, aid in the very least in the cure of gout, acute or chronic, unless a primary liver affection be its prime cause in the organopathic sense. Of course gout may further affect the liver and bowels as well as any other part ; what I mean is, that these do not necessarily conduce physiologically to the production of gout. And why I feel so satisfied of the relatively unimportant participation of the liver and intestine in the production of gout is because I have many times had to treat severe cases of gout in which purgation had been thoroughly carried out with no advantage whatever,

but rather the contrary; and, moreover, it is by no means an uncommon thing for very gouty people to
suffer from habitual looseness of
the bowels, and yet the gout does
not diminish. On the other hand,
as before remarked, I am strongly
of opinion that the spleen is very
intimately concerned in the production of gout.

There does not exist, to my
knowledge, any treatise on the
homoeopathic treatment of gout,
and the treatment of gout is, I believe, not the strongest point of
the homoeopathic school. This is
very likely not true of individual
homoeopathic practitioners, whose
successes in gout may have been
many and mighty; but speaking
generally, the homoeopathic *litera-*

ture of gout is not brilliant. And this I believe to be due to the fact that gout *is* very difficult to cure dynamically, because we have behind the symptoms the uric deposits ; and remedies that are homoeopathic to the symptoms of the gouty patients from the deposits are not necessarily homoeopathic to the state productive of such deposits ; and it must be manifest that remedies, to be really curative of arthritis, must be homoeopathic to the state productive of such deposits of urates within the tissues. It is not enough to cure the symptoms due to the urates : to be the remedy of the case, not only the uric deposits must be included within the simillimum, but the state which produces such deposits.

Whether any *one* remedy can be expected to be homoeopathic to the state productive of gouty doposits, and of such deposits themselves, may be a debatable point. The production of deposits of urates of sodium in pigeons by Ebstein and others by injections of bichromate of potassium is not what I mean exactly, for the gouty state takes time to be produced, and does not consist merely in the deposition of urate of sodium into the superacid tissues. However we here need more knowledge. It is just this point that has not received due attention in the homoeo-therapeutics of gout, and hence it has come to pass that our literature on the subject is so very poor. No doubt the clinical work of our school is better

than our hereto relative literature,
for some of our best clinicians do
not write ; still our literature ought
to be the register of our best work,
and in this register outsiders should
be able to find ample proofs that
the homoeopathic principle is use-
ful, and workable also in such a
substantive disease as gout in its
acute form. It is not enough to
affirm that the principle of similars
is workable : we must prove it ;
and this can be done.

Now, so long as I kept to the
ordinarily commended homoeopathic remedies for gout, so long
were my results mostly only tedious
recoveries ; cures they could not be
fairly called. One thing only could
I boast of in the simply symptomatic

homoeopathic treatment of gout : my patients recovered—slowly and tediously, it is true—but still they recovered *completely*, with undamaged constitutions and unharmed *organs*, and the gentle treatment not only ended thus in integral restitution, but subsequent attacks became milder and less frequent, so that even that was, I think, a fair record. But we can do more than that, as I will show. Not a few mighty men have expressed the opinion that the proper *role* of the physician is merely to pilot the patient from the sea of sickness into the harbour of health. Still, my own ambition is never satisfied with such a *role ;* my constant strivings are ever directed to being the master of disease, and I am not satisfied unless and until I deem myself the victor, always within the limitations of "thus far and no further."

In genuine gout we have to deal with the *attack :* this is the mountain of difficulty.

I was very early in my career warned against the use of *Colchicum* in the cure of gout, because of its deleterious effects on the kidneys. . . . "Rely upon *Colchicum* in gout, and you will get plenty of Bright's disease," was the advice to me given by a most experienced clear-headed physician and hence it has come to pass that I have myself no experience of *Colchicum* in gout, good or bad. I do not remember ever having prescribed it a single time. And hence the gouty onslaught has always been, for me, a difficult task. For there can be no doubt, judging by the clinical records of *Colchicum*, that of all known remedies used thus far, *Colchicum* has far and away the greatest influence over the gouty manifestations. My own suspicions are to the effect that *Colchicum* is homoeopathic to some of these external manifestations which it effectively gets rids of, but leaves the uric deposits in the blood and tissues. The outside symptoms are gone, the inside disease remains. Is it not an oft-told tale that "X. got the gout; he took *Colchicum* and was much relieved, but—he was later on seized with great pain in the chest and died."

Natrum muriaticum, 6 trit., has
helped me in some cases of acute
gout very satisfactorily ; the urine
thickened and deepened in color,
and the attack was broken up. It
is still used by me in gout pretty
considerably where prominent *Nat.
mur.* symptoms are present, and
specially where the patient has
taken much quinine, or is chilly, or
his gouty attack is apt to be stirred
up by a visit to the seaside. I use
6 grains of the 6th trituration
every two or three hours, and expect the urine to deepen in color
and thicken within two days simultaneously wherewith the gouty
manifestations usually abate. I
have no faith in gout cures unless
they thicken the urine. If the
heart is weak or atheromatous I

commonly rely on *Gold* : and it is a
veritable friend in need and indeed.
If the skin is fairly normal I use
the *Aurum muriaticum 3*, five drops
in a tablespoonful of water every
three or four hours. If the skin is
very wet and patient sweats unduly
I give *Aurum muriaticum natur-
atum 3*. in the same dose as the
simple muriate, and am generally
not disappointed with the results. I
have also used *Jaborandi* and its al-
kaloid *Pilocarpine* with good results.
In the treatment of acute gout it is
sound practice to keep an eye on
the stomach first, the heart next,
and collaterally on the reciprocal
relations, topographic and patho-
logic, of the heart and liver and
spleen respectively ; and this because the heart, with liver, spleen.

stomach, and kidneys, are really the "interested parties" in acute gout. When I speak of stomach I really mean the epigastrium and more precisely speaking, the solar plexus —to which aether, zincum, and hydrocyanic acid will bring prompt and efficient help.

Have we a remedy or remedies essentially Homœopathic to the gouty attack ?

To this I think an affirmative answer can now be given. I propose to show that *Urtica urens,* the common stinging nettle, is such a one, and I think *Natrum muriaticum* has strong claims to be so considered also. But *Nat. mur.* is a classic remedy in homoeopathy ; it is well known and much used by such as have gripped the true inwardness of homoeopathic drug-action. As I will presently relate, I have used *Urtica urens* a good deal for some years in ague and spleen affections, and thus it comes to pass that I have had ample opportunities of becoming intimately acquainted with its powers. Patients under the influence of small material doses of *Urtica* will often pass quantities of gravel. The first occasion of my observing this in a striking manner was in a middle-aged maiden lady, who came over from Germany to place herself under my care, who smelled so strongly of nettles that it nauseated me whenever it was my duty to examine her. She had, amongst many ailings, an enlarged spleen, and for this splenic enlargement I gave the mother tincture of *Urtica urens.* I was led to use it from the burning pains as well as the odour. This lady passed a very large quantity of gravel by the urine while under its influence. I did not attach very much importance to this, as patient was in the habit of passing considerable quantities of gravel *with her motions*, localised abdominal pain generally preceding such an occurrence by a number of days. She was in the habit of indicating a spot just under her spleen as her "gravel-pit." But when I observed others who, being under the influence of *Urtica urens*, passed grit and gravel pretty freely for the first time in their lives, I came to the

conclusion that the *Urtica* possesses
the power of eliminating the urates
from the economy.   And it slowly
became clear to my mind that *Urtica*
might be the very remedy I had
long been in quest of, viz., a quickly-
acting, easily-obtained homoeopathic remedy for the Attacks of
gout, or some of them, for of course
we, of experience, never expect uniform results any more than we expect all the trees in a forest to be of
the same height. I subsequently became aware that *Urtica urens* is
contingently capable of producing
fever, as some subsequent experience will show. The fever of the
gouty attack is not great, but still
feverishness *is* a part of such attacks, and I should not feel sure of
of the homoeopathicity of a remedy

thereto did it not possess the symptom "fever" in its pathogenesis.

I then proceded to employ the *Urtica urens* in the classic attacks of genuine gout, and that with very great satisfaction indeed. Within a few hours after beginning its use the urine becomes fairly free, of a high colour, and the bottom of the vessel is often found more or less covered with urates in the form of grit and gravel, and simultaneously herewith the gouty attack begins to subside.* I call the discovery, of this gravel-expelling power of *Urtica*, *great*; well, it has been *great* to me in my clinical work, and my patients are generally

---

*An allopathic neighbour tells me that *Urtica* was much used in olden times for gout—*nil nori sub sole !*

of the same opinion as myself,—so much so that one or two of the commercially minded among them have over and over again urged me to bring it out as my gout medicine; but I have no respect for nostrums or nostrum-mongers, and am quite content to make it known as a most valuable remedy in the treatment of acute gout, as it cuts short the attack *in a safe manner*, viz., by ridding the economy of the essence of the disease product, its actual suffering-producing material.

I call it a homoeopathic remedy because I believe it to be such, though it may be just an organopathic remedy and simply act as a splenic, for *Urtica* is undoubtedly a powerful splenic, as I have often clinically demonstrated. The

provings of *Urtica* have thus far
been only elementary, and its mode
of action has yet to be studied ; but
if time permit I will argue the point
at length later on.   It is my sheet-
anchor in both gout and gravel.   In
gravel it facilitates and accelerates
its passage, and ends by curing
the colic casually. My usual mode
of administering it is by giving 5
drops of the mother tincture in a
wineglassful of quite warm water,
frequently repeated, say every two
or three hours.   Only yesterday
morning I was called to see a gentleman 78 years of age suffering
from "his old enemy," viz , pains in
his left kidney region. I prescribed
Urtica every two hours, and called
again late in the evening. . . .
"Oh ! the pains is gone, and I have

passed a lot of gravel." In my practice this is an oft-told tale. In the treatment of gout and gravel it may be of importance to remember that the nettle is not an uncommon plant, and that nettle-tea acts just as well as the tincture of which I make use. The nettle is a very curious plant, that appears to follow man the world over. I have read that its original *habitat* is somewhere in Asia, whence supposedly started the wanderings of the peoples. As we all know, it dies down in the winter and shoots out again in the spring. Certain it is that it follows man wherever he goes. I lately inquired of a gentleman resident in Western Australia whether there was any nettle indigenous to that region, and received a reply to the effect that he knew of no Australian nettle, but that the English nettle sprang up everywhere near human habitations. Last year, when in the country for my holidays, I searched about to find out where the nettles best throve, and found that the plant was most flourishing in and at the sides of ditches which carried off the fluid sewage form the cottages, and thus possibly living to some extent on urinous food. This point is somewhat interesting and suggestive.

Story of the Nettle as a Medicine.

Although nothing to do with my present thesis, except in so far as it gives an account of my first acquaintance with the nettle as a medicine, I am nevertheless constrained to give a history of the nettle as a medicine in gout, ague-cake, and gravel; I mean, of course, my history of the nettle.

Twenty years ago I was treating a lady for intermittent fever of the mild English type, when one day my patient came tripping somewhat jauntily into my consulting-room and informed me that she was quite cured of her fever, and wished to consult me in regard to another matter. I at once turned to my notes of her case, and inquired more closely into the matter of the cure, in order to duly credit my prescribed remedy with the cure, and the more so as ague is not always easily disposed of therapeutically. "Oh !"

said the lady, "I did not take your medicine at all, for when I got home I had such a serve attack of fever that my charwoman begged me to allow her to make me some nettle-tea. as that was a sure cure of fever. I consented, and she at once went into our garden, where there are plenty of nettles growing in a heap of rubbish and brickbats, and got some nettles, of which she made me a tea, and I drank it. It made me very hot. The fever left me, and I have not had it since."

Homage to the charwoman of nettle-tea fame !

The thing escaped my mind for years, but one day being in difficulty about a case of ague, I treated with a tincture of nettles and cured it straight away, and my next case also, and my next, and almost every case ever since, and with very nearly uniform success. Some of my cases of ague cured with nettle-tincture were most serve ones, invalided home from India and Burmah. And quite lately a patient living in Siam, to whom I had sent a big bottle of nettle-tincture, wrote me :—"The tincture you sent us has very greatly mitigated the fever we get here. Please order us another bottle!" *Ague_Halfcold chill Spleen Enlarged*

I say *almost* every case has yielded to *Urtica urens* ; every case, of course, has not.

The gouty attack.

Two years since a middle-aged gentleman of position was down

with an attack of gout that had
relapsed over and over again, and
he had then been in and out of
these attacks for nearly six months.
He had been swamped with alkalies
and *Colchicum*, and mercilessly
purged and lulled with narcotics
most alarmingly. He thought he
would "try homoeopathy," and sent
for the writer. I put him on *Urtica
urens* as already described, and he
was out and about in a fortnight.
In a couple of days of the treatment his urine became dark, plenti-
ful, and loaded with uric acid gravel.
His enthusiasm knew no bounds,
and he declared that no remedy he
had ever taken (and he had had
attacks of gout over and over again,
and had taken pretty well all known
gout medicines) had really touched

his gout like the *Urtica*. With him
and his club intimates I became
known as Dr. Urtica.

A gentleman of 50 odd years of
age, now resident in London, consulted me for gout in the fall of the
year 1890. He had long lived in
India and suffered much from
malaria. After a few weeks of
Urtica, 10 drops in a wineglassful
of water night and morning, he was
free from gout, and "My diarrhoea
has gone, my gout also ; my
digestion is better than for long,
and my skin is much cleaner."

At the end of the year 1893 the
wife of a country square in North-
unberland wrote me in great haste

that her goodman was down with a
severe bout of gout, and would I
send him medicine forthwith. I
ordered him ten drops of the tincture three times a day, and this
rather large dose as he is a very big
man, of a somewhat thirsty disposition. I heard no more of the matter;
but three or four months later the
lady consulted me on her own
account here in London, and inci-
dentally remarked. "That medicine
soon cured my husband's gout, and
he has not had any since," As before remarked, there is fever with
the gouty attack, and a remedy to
meet it homoeopathically should
show its power of producing fever.
Urtica urens, in my hands, has
produced fever over and over again.
In most cases in which its admini-

stration was followed by febrile
symptoms there was, at least, an
antecedent history of malarialism,
or actually of recent or remote
ague, but this was not invariably
the case. Moreover the same thing
obtains in regard to China. Hahnemann had had ague before he
proved the bark on himself and
found out its fever-producing power,
on which such a huge superstruc-
ture has been so solidly erected,—
i. e., homoeopathy.

The pathogenetic fever of
Urtica urens.

On October 3, 1893, a mother of
a family, pretty strong, 42 years of
age, came under my care for flatulent dyspepsia. No hitory of ague

or malaria She complained of left
sided pain, with coldness and chilli
ness, which led me to prescribe
Urtica urens θ, 10 drops in water,
night and morning. She reported :
"I cannot go on with his medicine ;
it sets all my pulses beating, makes
me terribly giddy,* makes me feel
as if I were going to topple (for-
wards) in my bed, and then a bad
headache comes on, and when I
take it at night it makes me very
feverish, so I am leaving it off."

Just nine months later I saw
this lady, and inquired if she re-
membered the very first remedy
I gave her. "Oh ! yes ; it made
me terribly giddy, and when I took
it at night it brought on fever, so I

*I have several times cured vertigo with *Urtica*.—
J. C. B.

could not go on with it ; and, indeed, I still have some of it left at
home now." When she took the
Urtica in the morning she did not
observe that it caused any feverish
symtoms, only when she took
it at night. The fever of gout
generally comes on at night.

II.

A middle-aged Indian officer
suffering from Scinde boils consulted me at the end of September 1893
for said boils, that were growing
worse rather than better, although
he had been home on their account
on leave for five months. He received from me *Urtica* θ. 12 drops
in water night and morning,
because I regarded it as of malarial

3

nature, for he had had ague years
ago, and was still in the habit of
taking quinine off and on for fear
of its returning, since almost any
cold would bring it back. The
taking of the *Urtica* was followed
by a furious outburst of fever, so
severe that patient's condition
caused his friends considerable anx-
iety. He, however, made a quick
and complete recovery.

III.

Another case was also that of an
officer invalided home from India
suffering from "liver" and malarialism, and to whom I gave 10
drops of *Urtica urens* twice a day
for his general condition. This,
too, was followed with very severe

fever with unusually long stages, from which he recovered under *Natrum muriaticum*, 6 trituration, 6 grains every two hours. The subsequent report being—"Those powders cured the fever, but he was very much pulled down."

It is distinctly curious to note the remarkable effects of *Natrum muriaticum* and *Urtica urens* in gout, as well as in ague and malarialism.

Urate of Sodium in the Treatment of Gout.

I have used *Urea*, *Uric acid*, and *Urate of Sodium* in gout, and they are of distinct value ; they have helped me most and best where the deposits persist : they stir up the lazy deposits, so to speak, and help to eliminate them.

Daphne, *Mezereon* and *Physalis alkekengi* have been used by me in gout off and on with a certain amount of benefit. So have *Bryonia*, *Rhus*, *Pulsatilla*. and *Bacillinum*, and many others, each in its own sphere, in accordance with the indications and data of homoeopathic pharmacology, as well as with my own clinical experience. And *Aconite* has helped me up to a certain point many times : notably in the stiff-nesses that remain after gout, have I found *Aconite* 3^x or 3, given night and morning, of positive avail.

Bellis perennis does distinct good in the after-gout debility of the limbs; and *Cypripedium pubescens* (and also the powder *Cypripedinum* 3ˣ) is its equivalent in the sphere of the nerves in the after-gout adynamia and neurasthenia. Where there are actual calculi that require solution before they can be passed, *Piperazinum purum* bulks up very imposingly, and I think no therapeutist can afford to ignore it after the record following. I take it from the *Therapist*, July 14. 1894 :—

"An Aggravated Case Of Nephritic Calculi Successfully Treated With Piperazine

By S. W. C. Brown, Surgeon to Trinidad Hospital, Colorado.

"The author having been a sufferer from nephritic calculi dur-

ing the past seven years, and
helped at last by *Piperazine* after
all other remedies had been tried
without relief, brings his own case
before the profession in the somewhat deficient state of literature.

"His trouble commenced about
seven years ago with a sudden
attack of nephritic colic, accompanied by the passage of urate
crystals, so sharply defined and so
numerous that the mucous mem-
brane was cut by them. They
increased in number until half a
teaspoonful was passed with each
evacuation of the bladder, generally
accompanied by haematuria. The
body-weight at this time was 260
lbs., urine of normal specific gravi-
ty, containing pus corpuscles, blood,

and epithelial cells. Shortly after this attack eight calculi were passed, five being unusually large, and all exceedingly painful, unconsciousness supervening in the case of four from three to fifteen hours.

"During the past seven years every sudden jar or jolt produced intense pain over the region of the left kidney, and although eighteen months ago the symptoms suddenly ceased for a time on taking *Herba delvey*, a local remedy of great repute amongst the Mexicans, they return again within three months, whilst during the treatment an enlarged prostate and exceedingly irritable bladder were probably due to the remedy.

"In October last a very violent haemorrhage took place from the bladder or kidney, continuing for four weeks with intense pain, constant catheterisation being required. The incessant pain was localised over the left kidney, and necessitated a hypodermic injection of 8 grains *morphia* daily.

"About this time the author's attention was called to *Piperazine*, although having been on all sorts of treatment without relief, he was rather sceptic as to its value, and did not take to it very readily. The condition was then—weight 170 lbs., pulse 60, profuse diaphoresis, very feeble, confined to bed ; examination of urine showed pus, albumen, blood, only 9 ounces daily, which required to be drawn off by catheter, and large amounts of urates.

"The author commenced taking 15 grains *Piperazine* daily in one quart of water. On the third day the urine had increased to 39 ounces, and continued to gain in quantity until the normal quantity was reached, which has continued to the present time. The most satisfaction was, however, afforded by the fact that on the fourth day the intense pain began to grow less, and continued to do so until it entirely ceased. The *Morphia* was gradually decreased, and *Phenocoll hydrochloride* in 10-grain doses taken in its place. At the present time weight is increasing at the rate of 4 lbs. per week, appetite is very good, urine perfectly normal, and business capability restored. The urine examined from time to time whilst under *Piperazine* treatment showed the passage of excessive quantities of urates, but they were always in solution and gave no trouble in voiding.

'In conclusion, *Piperazine* has certainly shown itself in this case a very prompt and powerful solvent of uric acid calculi, and one of very great value in those cases where the knife has hitherto been of doubtful value. (*Notes on New Remedies*)."

It is true that weighty men declare that *Bicarbonate of soda* is more than equal to *Piperazine*, but

this I much doubt.   However, I
have no intention of dealing ex-
haustively with all the gout remedies, but merely glance at the
outer world just to see what they
are doing and thinking in regard
to gout.   And having, so to speak,
gone round the show, I find but
very little progress, if any, in the
old school's ways of thinking and
acting.   That is to say, the morbid
product of the disease only is regarded, the *patient* is lost sight of.
Thus we find matters stand at the
Eleventh   International   Medical
Congress,   held   in   Rome,   1894.
Dr. C. Mordhorst, of Wiesbaden,
there read a paper entitled "Die
bei der Behandlung der Gicht und
Harnsäureconcremente in Betracht
kommenden   Mittel   und   ihre

Wirkungsweise," and there defines
gout as *the uric acid diathesis*,
and the gist of the whole thing
consists in using alkalies to render
the superacid gouty ones alkaline !
Here we again stumble against the
fundamental principle of curative
medicine,—Whether are diseases
best treated by contraries or by
similars ? That the gouty do beyond question derive *temporary*
benefit from *Piperazine* and the
alkaline treatment admits of no
manner of doubt; they render the
superacid fluids of the organism for
the time being alkaline, whereby
the superacidity is got rid of and
a transitory cure is effected ; but
the cure is ephemeral only, it does
not last.

Mordhorst says (p. 25)—"The

only question to consider in the
effective treatment of the uric acid
diathesis is to render the fluids
of the body as alkaline as possible."
Now this I deny absolutely. It is
not possible to cure the uric acid
diathesis with alkalies, inasmuch as
the alkalescence thus produced is
only the chemical, and not vital ; as
for the alkalescence thus set up, to
be rendered permanent it is requi-
site to continue unceasingly the input of alkalies. This Mordhorst
himself admits, and, indeed, proves ;
and the *raison d' etre* of his paper
at the International Congress is the
recommendation of the Weisbaden
Gichtwasser, which he says is the
best of all anti-arthritic waters.
And what is this best of all anti-
gout waters capable of effecting ;

Let Dr. Mordhorst answer (p. 46):
—"The more *Gichtwasser* is
drunk the sooner the sufferings are
relieved ; if as much as three
bottles are daily consumed, it takes
from three to five weeks before
amelioration sets in ; if only one or
two bottles are daily drunk, it may
take months to get rid of the
sufferings, but eventually all the
troubles disappear, and this condition remains permanent so long
as the prescribed mode of life is not
too often sinned against, *and from
half a bottle to a bottle of the water
be daily drunk*" *!!* This is positive and honest : after the best
anti-gout treatment by mineral
waters and alkalies *plus* dietetic
and mode-of-life modifying restrictions, the permanent condition is

one of ever-continuing restrictions, and daily drinking of mineral water.

Dr. Mordhorst is himself very gouty, and he gives his own case as one cured by the Wiesbaden *Gichtwasser* (pp. 48—9), and he thus describes his own case :—

"I belong to a very gouty family. My father suffered, my three sisters still suffer from gout. An elder brother of mine died at the age of 46 years of uric acid renal calculi. Already four or five years ago I at times felt a painful sensation on pressure in my left leg along the course of the sciatic nerve. About a year and a half ago I discovered on the inner side of my left knee several small tophi, which at times pain on pressure, and incon-

venience me in walking. I have also
discovered gouty nodes in several
other parts of my body, but these
are but seldom in evidence. Whenever I get pains in these affected
parts, I drink, for four or five days,
two to three bottles of *Gichtwasser*
every day, to get rid of them. The
urine becomes strongly, and the
cutaneous secretions faintly, alkaline. A small gouty tophus in the
flexor pollicis longus of my left
thumb, that remained from a slight
acute attack, disappeared, all but
slight traces, after a prolonged
course of the *Gichtwasser*."

Note well that this is the *cured*
state.

It must, therefore, be manifest
that the mineral water, the alkaline

treatment of gout (and the piperazine cure must be reckoned to the
alkaline) is a cure, more or less,
of the *gouty products*, but has little
or no influence upon the gout
disease itself in the sense of the
uric acid *diathesis*. The products
are got rid of; the *power of producing* remains unimpaired. The
grit, gravel, tophi, and, with *Piperazine*, perhaps even calculi, can be
eliminated by the chemical treatment, but the diathesis remains
untouched.

But do I maintain that when the
gouty attack is got rid of with the
aid of *Urtica* or *Natrum muriaticum*
or other homoeopathic remedies,
do I maintain that the uric acid
diathesis is mended ?

No, I do not altogether. What
I do, however, maintain, is that
after this treatment the attacks of
gout are milder and much less
frequent ; but whether this greater
mildness and infrequency be due
to the influence of the remedies
exclusively, or to the greater subsequent care in living, is not easily
determined. Perhaps a little of both.

Earlier on in these pages I said
that gout, for me, is the smoke and
soot of the organism, resulting from
its combustive activities : this is, of
course, a figure of speech ; my real
meaning is practically identical
with the data of science in regard to
the uric acid diathesis. Only I part
company with scholastic physicians
where they stick fast at the uric acid
deposits and their accompanying

super-acid state,—these are, indeed, my "smoke and soot," but neither is the ailment itself. The gouty individual is like a smoky chimney: his organism does the carrying-off imperfectly, and as in the case of the smoky chimney it does not suffice to get the sweeps, but the services of a chimney-doctor are needed to remedy the defect, so in the gouty person this uric acid may be got rid of by *Gichtwasser, alkalies, Piperazine* or *Urtica,* but the real cure has not been effected ; the smoke and soot only have been cleared away, the products are gone, the power of further production remains ; only the sweep has done his work not the chimney-doctor; he it is whose services have now to be invoked.

Differences Between the Cure of the Gouty State by Mineral Water and Alkalies and by Homœopathic Remedies.

Essentially the cure of the gouty state by mineral waters and alkalies is mainly chemical, viz., they set up a condition of alkalescence, and the uric concretions are thus rendered soluble, and the mass of fluid drunk washes them out, while in the homoeopathic treatment *the organism itself becomes its own sweep and turns them out.* In the former case the urine becomes clear, while under the homoeopathic action of the remedies the urine becomes *dark* and *visibly charged with gravel.* This difference is essentially great and important, for while both end in the washing out of the deposits, the same begin forthwith to accumulate almost as soon as the remedies are left off; on the other hand, under the homoeopathic remedies the organism has itself done the work, and at least a certain time elapses before new deposits take place, so that one has time to enter upon a real cure of the diathesic quality. Only in the case of large portions of gravel, and in the case of actual calculi, does the *Piperazine* and *Gichtwasser* treatment seem to me to be preferable, inasmuch as in this latter case the organism itself cannot possibly do the work until the concretions have been dissolved. In ordinary manifestations of gout it is the organism itself that requires to be called up homoeopathically to do its own work ; usually there are no concretions of any great size present, as, for instance, in the acute attack of gout. I have previously stated that Homoeopathic literature, so far as it is known to me, has not won any great laurels in the matter of gout. Moreover, I formerly felt the homoeopathic treatment of gout to be very tedious and unsatisfactory, and now I will proceed to explain why that has heretofore been the case ; at least, so it seemed to me.

The True Homœo-Therapeutics of Gout.

In a given case of gout the symptoms are not those of the

individual himself, but of the gouty matter, of its material presence in the individual : the pain, the swelling, the redness, the tenderness, the fever, the restlessness—these are produced by the gouty material, which we see from the fact that they disappear as soon as this material is washed out ; so that what we require are remedies that are homoeopathic to the state of the patient which preceded the gouty deposit into the tissues, inclusive of these deposits. In fact, the pathology of gout must be considered, in prescribing adequately, homoeopathically. Our anti-arthritic remedies must be capable of producing a state that leads up to a deposit of gouty material, and not be merely homoeopathic to the symptoms produced by the material itself. The process, together with the product, must be within the pathogenesis, or else a real totality of the symptoms is not obtained. In fine, the gouty material is the *stop-spot* of the action of the remedies thus far mostly employed in the homoeopathic treatment of gout. I have been severely taken to task for claiming that pathology must be considered in a homoeopathic prescription in order to ascertain the *stop-spot* of the action of each remedy, but I beg these esteemed colleagues to note that I did not say *morbid anatomy*, but *pathology*, two widely different things. Morbid anatomy we study in the deadhouse; that may or may not have to be considered as throwing some light on a given subject, but pathology is the doctrine of the disease in the living,—the actual pathic biology of the diseased individual, which *ends* where the morbid anatomy *begins*. Do my esteemed colleagues really mean that this pathic biology of the patient enters not into the homoeopathic equation?

I trow not.

Attack Of Gout Cured By *Urtica Urens.*

Lord X. had an attack of gout three years ago, and it fell to my lot to treat him for it. It was the classic podagra. I gave *Urtica urens* θ, five drops in a wineglassful of warm water, every three hours, and his lordship was about as usual in

4

ten days. In another attack since
then the same remedy acted with
equal promptitude, and to the
patient's great satisfaction. His
lordship has had quite a number of
attacks of gout, and has had the
advantage of the services of the
very greatest authorities on gout,
in London, and, moreover, he has
been to the leading spas for gout,
and hence his opinion is of value,
and this runs thus—"I have never
taken any remedy that has done so
much for me as *Urtica*; there is no
doubt about that."

Gouty Ophthalmia.

A very gouty city gentleman,
just turned 50 years of age, came on
21st October, 1892, to consult me

for a slight attack of gouty ophthalmia of his left eye. I ordered *Urtica urens* θ ten drops in water, night and morning, and this cured the ophthalmia within a week, amelioration setting in already within twenty-four hours. I have been in the habit of seeing this gentleman for a number of years for gouty manifestations, amongst which was a very obstinate gouty eczema.

Dr. Holtz* maintains that the fever of gout, as observed by him in hundreds of cases, rarely exceeds about half a degree, whereas the fever of rheumatism commonly runs high, and this he regards as an

---

*Das. Wesen und die hygienische Behandlung der Gicht. Detmold. 1894.

essential difference between the two processes. This is, no doubt, correct ; still there *is some* fever, and at times there are distinct rigors. There is often, as Tanner points out, uneasiness in the left rib region, with inability to lie on that side, so that, with this symptom added, I think I may fairly claim that *Urtica* is a true simile to gout.

It has—

1. Fever, heat and cold, flushes.
2. Passage of girt and gravel.
3. Uneasiness of left rib region.
4. Great restlessness.

We will now go on to the next point in the treatment of gout. That much of the gout we meet with is more or less produced by alcohol, is amply manifest. It

becomes, therefore, a question worth
considering whether the effects of
alcohol *per se* can be homoeopathically antidoted, and if so, by what
remedies.

On a Remedy Homœopathically Antidotal to The Effects of Alcohol.

For some years past I have been
acquainted with a remedy that
antidotes the effects of alcohol very
prettily, as I will now proceed to
show. I enter upon the subject in
this place, because it deserves to be
made widely known, and also because, in the treatment of gout,
the alcoholism not infrequently
bars the way. The remedy I refer
to is the distilled spirit of acorns—

Spiritus glandium quercus. My
first account of it will be found in
my "Diseases of the Spleen,"
where this *Spiritus glandium quercus*
is dealt with as a spleen medicine.
I speak of set purpose of the homoeopathic antidote, because alcoholism
is a disease, and as such must be
met by specific medication.

Some of Rademacher's patients
complained to him that while taking
his acorn medicine they felt in
their heads somewhat as if they
were drunk ; but as Rademacher
did not believe in the law of
similars—indeed, knew but little
about it— their complaint had no
ulterior significance to him, but
still it struck him as worthy of
record ; and he accordingly did

record it in the following words
(see *Erfahrung sheillehre*, p. 209, i.)
:—"Einige, aber wenige Menschen,
bemerken gleich nach dem Ein-
nehmen ein eigenes, kaum eine
oder zwei Minuten anhaltendes
Gefuhl im Kopfe, welches ange-
blich der Berauschung aehlich sein
soll." Turned into English :—"A
few, but not many, of those who
take it, immediately feel a peculiar
sensation in the head, which they
say is like they feel when they are
drunk, the sensation lasting only a
minute or two." Now, in the light
of the homoeopathic law this symptom is eminently suggestive, but
whether anyone besides myself has
ever noticed this symptom I am
not aware. But it made a lasting
impression on my mind years ago.

Redemacher had previously related the following brilliant cure.
. . . He says that in order to get a clear idea of the action of the remedy, he caused to be prepared a tincture of acorns, of which he gave a teaspoonfull in water five times a day to an almost moribund brandy toper, who had long been suffering from a spleen affection, that at times had caused him a good deal of pain, and who, at the time in question, had severe ascites, and whose lower extremities were dropsical up as far as the knees. Our author was of opinion that the affection was a primary disease of the spleen, and reasoned that if the tincture of acorns cured the spleen, the kidneys would duly resume work, and the ascitic and

anasarcous state would disappear.
He soon found he was right;
patient at once began to pass more
urine, but he complained that every
time he took a dose of the medicine
he got a constriction of the chest,
and this Rademacher ascribed to
the astringent quality of the acorns,
and to avoid this he had the
tincture of acorns *distilled*. The ad-
ministration of this distilled preparation was not followed by any un-
pleasent symptom, the quantity of
urine passed increased still more,
the tension in the praecordia slowly
lessened, and this inveterate drunkard got quite well, much to the
amazement of everybody, Rademacher included, for he did not at
all expect him to recover.

Now, it must be admitted that a remedy that can cure an old drunkard of general dropsy and restore him to health deserves closer acquaintance. And when we regard it from the pathogenetic side as producing, of course, contingently, a cephalic state resembling alcoholic intoxication, and then from the clinical side as having cured an abandoned drunkard, it lookes very much as if we had a remedy homoeopathic to alcoholism. I may add that Rademacher nowhere hints that the *Spiritus glandium quercus* stands in any relation to alcoholism ; he regards it merely as a spleen medicine, specially indicated in dropsy due to a primary speen affection. At first, I regarded it merely in the same light; but when I really gripped the significance of the pathogenetic symptoms just quoted, I thought we might find in our common acorns a notable homoeo-pathic anti-alcoholic.

Now let me give some of my clinical experience on this point, so that my readers may be able to judge for themselves whether this be so.

The *Spiritus glandium quercus* Homœopathically Antidotal To The Ill Effects of Alcohol.

I. Observation.

Colonel X., aged 64, came under my observation on January 15, 1889, broken down with gout and chronic

alcoholism, and pretty severe bron-
chitis. Heart's action irregular ;
liver and spleen both enlarged ; and
he complained bitterly of a gnaw-
ing in the pit of the stomach. His
gait was unsteady and tottering, his
hands quivered, and altogether he
was in a sorry plight. The poor
fellow had lost his wife, and had for
a good while tried to rub along
with the aid of a little Dutch
courage, in the shape of nips of
spirits, for which he was always
craving. Severe windy spasms ;
no sugar, no albumen.

℞ *Spiritus glandium quercus* θ,
10 drops in water, three times a day.

January 22.—On this day—a
week from his first visit—he walked
briskly into my consulting room,

and brightly exclaimed, "Well, I think you have worked a miracle;" and the curious thing was that his craving for spirits was notably less, he having consumed only one-third of a bottle of whisky in the week, instead of two bottles, which was his usual allowance. The windy spasms had ceased, and his foul breath had become sweet; and finally, his spleen had gone down in size very notably. To leave off the *Quercus*.

February 5.—So little craving for whisky that he offers to leave it off; much less phlegm in chest; no spasms; altogether quite a different man, but is depressed.

℞ *Spiritus glandium quercus* θ, 7 drops in water, three times a day.

February 19.—He is chirpy again, and has no craving for whisky.

The remedy was repeated in May, and I learned some months afterwards, from his daughter, that the colonel continued in fair health, and partook of stimulants "like other people," and without any "craving."

II. Observation.

A London merchant, 57 years of age, came under my care on October 16, 1888, for necrosis of all the nails of his right hand, and most of those of the left hand, and of nearly all his toe-nails ; severe arcus senilis, rushes of blood to the head, buzzing in both ears. I discharged him cured at the end of the summer of 1891, so that he was under my very careful treatment for nearly three years. He was a candid, dutiful patient, and had his reward in being really and radically cured. He first had *Vanadium* 5, 5 drops in water, night and morning, and after one month of this his arcus senilis had notably diminished, and "I do not get so tried, and my hands do not tremble so much." The *Vanadium* was continued for a second month. "Much better in himself; can now do a day's work; trembling all gone; noises nearly well of the left ear, no better of the right." *Thuja* and many remedies followed, with steady amelioration, but something

seemed to bar the way to a perfect
cure, when he confessed that he
thought he took too much sherry
in nips. Like the colonel, he was
never intoxicated,—never, in fact,
morally intoxicated, but still never
free from the effects of his nips.

℞ *Spiritus glandium quercus* θ, 10
drops in water, night and morning.

This brought out a good deal of
gouty eczema of scalp, poll, and
backs of hands. It took me ten
months to really cure this eczema,
and then I had him back to the
Quercus, which he took, altogether,
for three months ; and then I find,
at the end of my record of his case
in my case-book the word . . .
well.

III. Observation.

The wife of an officer of position wrote to me some two years ago— ". . . I am not at all satisfied with my husband's appearance. We have had a shooting party, and I am sure he drinks too much. I can always tell by the look of his eyes ; they are so yellow, and puffy underneath. I wish you would send him something to put him right ; he says he is all right, but I am sure he is not, from his breath.

After a month of *Quercus,* I heard this : ". . . My husband looks wonderfully well."

IV. Observation.

A noble Nimrod, about 40 years
of age, a very free liver, and plagued
with attacks of gout, came under
my observation in the spring of
1891 for varicose veins of the lower
extremities, starting originally, it
seemed to me, from an enlarged
spleen, which was seemingly left
after typhoid fever. Knowing his
mode of life, and on account of the
spleen, I gave him *Quercus* for a
month, 10 drops at bedtime, and
then noted : "He likes his medicine,
as it keeps his bowels very regular."

May 15, 1891—Veins better ;
fewer rings under his eyes.

℞ *Petroleum* 5.

July 22.—"He feels his feet hot, and would like the first medicine (*Quercus*), as it seemed to make him feel so well.

℞ *Spiritus glandium quercus* θ, 10 drops in water, at bedtime.

September 8.—In rude health.

V. Observation.

The following case is very striking, and greatly impressed me :—

A country squire, from the shire of Moonrakers, bachelor, 60 years of age, was accompanied to me on October 3, 1893, by his brother, resident in London. This gentleman was so very ill that his case was regarded as quite hopeless. He was not capable of stating his own case, and hence his brother did it for him. Patient was flushed, and in much pain over the eyes and in both rib regions. Stooping caused very great pain, worse in the left hypochondrium. Both liver and spleen notably enlarged. He is exceedingly nervous, very depressed, glum, taciturn, and moved to tears by almost anything. He could not walk without spport, on account of his great giddiness. His breath was in the highest degree disgustingly stercoraceous (*merdeux*), so much so that I very nearly vomited when examining him. He was personally unknown to me, and I had no history of him, but that smell of breath is an unmistakable sign of the chronic tippler. I subsequently ascertained that he was quite a sober-living man, but took frequent nips, particularly when confined to the house by wet weather. But quite apart from this, the *Quercus* was manifestly homoeopathic to the case.

1. pain in the left side.
2. Giddiness.
3. Flushed state.

So I ordered *Spiritus glandium quercus* θ, 10 drops in water, three times a day.

October 10—Less fluttering; giddiness a little better; the tenderness of the rib region much diminished; *breath normal* !

He returned home in six weeks perfectly well. A prettier directart cure I think I have never seen.

VI. Observation.

Three months ago a city magnate, about 70 years of age, came to me for giddiness, flatulent dyspepsia depression of spirits, a flushed face, and "altogether below par." His conjunctivae were yellowish, his tongue foul, and his breath the same as in the last-narrated case—stercoraceous and nauseous. Under the *Quercus* the patient made a rapid recovery, his breath becoming sweet within four days. This stercoraceous smell is pathognomonic of undigested alcohol in the *primævæ*, and is readily perceived two yards away from the patient's mouth, and quite unbearable within a foot or two. Where this smell is present, there is no

need to make irritating inquiries as
to the imbibitionary habits of the
individual,—*Quercus* is indicated.
It does not, of course, follow that
the *Quercus* is indicated only in the
alcoholic state. I have used it in
the case of total abstainers where
giddiness and spleen trouble co-
exist. I name this lest I prejudice
the legitimate use of *Quercus*,
and motive it by narrating the
following little episode :—

Years ago I was attending the
wife of a certain bishop, Lady
Sarah X. She had incipient melig-
nant disease of the tongue, and
while inspecting the part I recalled
to my mind the experience of
Baron Storck and the state of his
tongue, and that of his famulus.

At the time I knew next to nothing of homoeopathic literature, and in my naivety I prescribed *Conium* for Lady Sarah. On my next visit I found her ladyship in a fearful tantrum, and, on inquiring, she screeched at me—"I have not taken your medicine, not a single drop of it."

"Why not ?"

"Why not, indeed ? It is *Conium*, and you prescribed it because I am and old women ! "

In vain I protested.*

---

*To the uninitiated I may explain that in the homoeopathic "little books" it is stated *under Conium* that it is good for the complaints of old women.

Does the Action of the *Spiritus glandium quercus* Extend to The Liquor Habit.

I think I must answer this very largely, though not entirely, in the negative. Its action antidotes the alcoholic state promptly and effectively, and the craving is at times greatly lessened, and in here and there a case cured altogether ; but speaking broadly, it stops short of the liquor habit. Just as *Urtica urens* will not cure the gouty disposition, except in a small degree, only helping the organism to cast out the gouty product itself, and so leaving it strengthened, so the *Glandes quercus* will not cure the liquor habit beyond a very limited degree. But inasmuch as the *Urtica* gets rid of the uric acid through and by the organism, so it is a homoeopathic remedy, and not either chemical, mechanical, or allopathic. And this is seen from the fact that an attack of gout got rid of by the aid of *Urtica* does *not* return so readily as when got rid of chemically through the artificial productions of alkalescence of the juices. That the action of *Urtica* is vital may be further seen from the fact that it by and by loses its action as the individual ceases to react to its stimulus, whereas the chemical cure can be repeated almost at will in the same individual. And reverting now for a moment to the influence of the *Glandes quercus* in the liquor habit : although it does not touch this where the habit is autochthonous, still where the habit is a liking for drink produced by drink purely and simply, and thus not autochthonous, but foreign, I have found that it does reach even the liquor habit itself. Thus in the case of the colonel which I have narrated, the *Spiritus glandium quercus did cure the liquor habit.* And how so? Surely it might be said, your distilled spirit of acorns either does, or does not, cure the liquor habit. It is in this wise : the colonel had no initially autochthonous liquor habit ; his wife died, and he began to nip out of loneliness ; when the action of one nip was on the wane a new nip followed, and so on in a circle. With the lapse of time that lonesomeness

became less ; time had caused the
wound to heal up, or, at any rate,
to skin over, but the drink-begotten
habit of drinking remained. The
acorn spirit cured the effect of the
drinking, *i. e.*, the acquired liquor
habit ; to this it is homoeopathic,
but it is *not* homoeopathic to the
liquor habit when due to other
causes (such as when a symptom of
consumptiveness, as it often is), and
will therefore not reach the habit,
but only the effects of the habit
around the alcohol. It is very
necessary to iterate and reiterate
this point, viz., what I have else-
where termed the *stop-spot* of
homoeopathic influence (see the pre-
liminary chapter in my *Curability
of Tumours by Medicine*). I per-
ceive our critics have not touched

upon this, but here and there a thinker has gripped the idea. It is difficult, somewhat abstruse, and takes a little time to filter through the mind and come out clear. I do not, as some aver, think little of symptoms or of symptomatology. What I say is this : We must not only take the symptoms and cover them ; we must also take the whole pathology, both of the disease and of the drug, and juxtapose the two processes, and then get in behind the symptoms and see whether in addition to the symptomatic similarity there is also coincidence of the drug pathology with the disease pathology, both running from start to goal. The reason why *Urtica* cannot cure the gout disease, but can only cure the gouty attack, is because its pathology goes only up to the product, and stops short of the production.

In regard to the question as to whether and how far the *Spiritus glandium quercus* reaches the craving for drink, the following letter from the wife of a gentleman to whom I had sent the remedy, is of a certain interest :—

"Dear Dr. Burnett,—To begin with my husband. He took the drops for a week, and then, as he caught a chill and was very poorly, and in the doctor's hand, I stopped the drops until he was a little better. He has now finished them about three weeks. He says his feet are not half so tender, and he can

walk with more ease and comfort.
He has not been feeling very well,
rather limp, and tired easily. He
has, however, slept well and quietly,
and while he was taking the drops
he drank less, both with and before
his meals. The last week or so he
is again taking sherry before meals
and beer at meal time, so I fully
expect a bilious attack, especially
as he is not as sweet-tempered as
usual. He has been eating better
and has come to bed earlier. He
has had B. and S. in the morning
before breakfast. So please do
give him something to stop this
craving for pick-me-ups. Air and
exercise he has in plenty, so if only
his craving, sinking feelings for
something can be stopped, he would
be as well as possible. I think his

hands look less swollen ; they were decidedly swollen a little while ago. He looks a little yellow in the eyes, and the skin a little dry and wrinkled. We all notice that he drinks less than he used to, and are all thankful for that ; so in time, perhaps, he will be quite right."

The Cod-Liver Oil Cure for Gout.

In the early part of this century, cod-liver oil was, in many parts of Europe, the most common cure for gout amongst the people, so it is highly probable that it has some therapeutic virtue in painful affections of the extremities. And since then it has been revived by the Faculty, and has again gone out of fashion. I know of no indications for its use, and though I have never ordered its use in gout, I have occasionally consented to its being used.

The Hot-Water Cure of Cadet De Vaux.

The cure of gout by drinking quantities of hot water was much in vogue in the early part of this century, and it has been revived again within the past few years, and at the present time is again much in vogue. It went out of fashion long ago, because of its real or supposed ill-effects upon the constitution. So far as my own experience goes, the hot-water treatment is indicated in the aged, and in those whose tissues are tough, dry,

and cold. In the young and middle-
aged, in the tender and in the
sappy, the hot-water treatment is
distinctly harmful. It attacks and
hurts the tender tissues, and may
not be used by the young at all.
The middle-aged may use it
occasionally, when there is much
acid in the intestines, and digestion
is at a standstill. At the present
time, the Salisbury treatment—
living on hot water and finely
minced meat—is quite the rage,
notably since a noble duke has
stood godfather to it. So far as I
have been able to judge, it is only
a disagreeable way of starving.
A lady tried it for some time—
I think seven weeks—and from
being a comely person, only somewhat stout, yet in full vigour, she

lost most of her flesh and all her
strength, and the uterine tumour,
for which the treatment was under-
taken, alone throve, and waxed
greater ; the patient herself became
so weak that she frequently fainted.
She was unable to stand from
weakness, and would certainly
have died had it not been given
up. The case was observed by
myself, and is not heresay. I know
a gentleman, about 50 years of age,
who has been doing the Salisbury
treatment for some months past ;
he is naturally thin and wiry, and
he is very enthusiastic about the
cure, although he confesses that
he is very weak, and can only just
drag himself slowly about. He
adopted the treatment for oxaluria
and great depression of spirits, and

maintains that he now passes no
oxalates, and is light-hearted, and
feels wonderfully well, so far as his
feelings go, notwithstanding the
bodily debility. "The Salisbury
treatment," said he to me the other
day, "is a grand thing to get rid of
all superfluous tissue." Of course ;
no one questions that we all can
get rid of our tissues by starvation.
The art is to *keep* plenty of good
tissues, and therewith remain in
good health and vigour. I have
tried many dietetic experiments
on myself, and thus have often
lessened and increased my bulk
almost at will, and what I have
invariably found is this : you cannot
make *big* fire with a *small* quantity
of fuel ; that is impossible. Consume,
as a general thing, very little, and

you can only spend a very little in energy ; you cannot get much out of little. Of course, you may get too bulky, and thus waste much energy in mere locomotion. That is a question of being overweighted ; and when some of this overweight is got rid of by diet, there is, apparently, more energy developed on less food, but this is only apparent and not real. For here we have two factors to consider :— First, the overweight is lessened, and less energy is required for locomotion ; and, secondly, the overweight that is got rid of must be *added* to the food taken, inasmuch as the dieted individual has himself consumed a portion of himself : his organism has used up some of its stored fat. But if the diminished

import of food be continued too
long, deterioration and debility
must ensue. This is where the
fallacy comes in stored food is used,
and so the quantity of fuel is *not*
less, whereas the bulk to be carried
is less, and so the initial state of the
spare diet process is very commonly
accompanied by a feeling of well-
being and lightness ; they feel so
much lighter, and get about so
much more easily. Of course they
do. But as soon as the stored-up
food is gone, weakness supervenes
if a too spare diet be persisted in.
Therefore, in all dieting we must
stop a little before the fatty reserve
store is all used up ; for if we go
on we just consume ourselves
and as far as this goes it is death.
This brings us along to the question

of diet in gout and diet for the fat. Fat people are not necessarily gouty, and gouty people are not necessarily fat : still gout and obesity touch one another so closely that they in a certain number of cases, are not easily separated in practice.

Let us consider, first, *food and work*, and then *height and weight*.

Food And Work.

In considering the question of diet we rarely find people take due cognizance of the mode of life of the individual who is to be fed, and yet in the case of horses, for instance, every horse-keeper feeds his horses according to what he expects them to do. I formerly, very frequently, went to a country house, four miles from the railway station, to see a patient suffering from a grave malady. For some weeks the ordinary carraige horses were sent to take me to the patient's abode, and so long as this was the case the hills offered no impediment, and I found myself transported rapidly ; and this was very satisfactory to me, for doctor's time is his capital. Patient's malady was, as before stated, a grave one, and his belongings were very anxious to get me to the house as quickly as possible, so good-conditioned horses were put in to the carriage. But after a while patient got better, and then I found that fat old pony was sent to the station to meet me, and it took us nearly an hour to reach the squire's mansion. On the way back to the station I inquired of the coachman how it was that "Shaggy" seemed so pumped out with such a short journey. Said he : "Well, you see, Sir, she is out at grass in the home-park, and gets no oats or dry food at all."

Now, the coachman's explanation of "Shaggy's" weakness gives us the clue to what I desire to say in regard to diet in general. When anyone asks—What am I to eat and drink ? the answer must duly reckon with the mode of life of the questioner, and the amount of work which is required of him. As a rule, no work whatever was required of "Shaggy :" she just ran about in

the home-park, thriving beautifully
on grass and water and on this diet
she seemed exceedingly happy and
plump and sleek, and when spoken
to would gallop away in fine style,
the picture of health, strength, and
happiness.   Yet   a   three   or four
miles', run, in a very light cart, was
a severe trial for "Shaggy." It is
not different with human beings ; if
they do nothing but just loll about—
turned out to grass, so to speak—
bread and water, with fruit and
vegelables, amply suffice ; but if
they work, they need the equivalent
of oats and dry food. I am here not
giving expression to mere theory,
for I have tried numerous experiments on my own person and
proved the point over and over
again ; and I emphatically affirm

that you cannot get much work out
of little food, any more than you
can make a very big fire with a
very little fuel. Whether the
authority be Salisbury, Canter-
bury, or York, I care not, you
cannot get *much* work out of a
spare *diet*.

And now as to

Height And Weight.

I go a little out of my way to
point out the common fallacy under-
lying almost all the data given as
to what the normal weight of a person of a given height should be. If
my reader will consult the tables, he
will find that the assumed basis is
faulty in a very important particular. Let me explain. Place a dozen

persons of a given height—say 5 fit.
9 in.—side by side in a row, and
as they are all the same height,
the tops of their heads will be in a
line, *but* their hips will be at a very
different heights. In fact, it will be
seen that the height of an individual is no sure guide to his *bulk*, and
therefore not to his weight. In
some a *long neck* makes an inch or
more difference, in others it is a
very long *thigh bone* that gives the
greater height ; but in both cases
the weight is not determined by the
length of the neck or of the legs,
but rather by the relative *length of
the trunk.*

There are many *big* people who
stand at 5 ft. 6 in., and there are a
good many *small* people who stand
about 6 feet high.

There is a saying amongst the people that little women make the best mothers ; but these so-called little women are really *big* women, only they are on *short legs*. When examined very closely I find they are large in the trunk and have fine pelves, while *big* women (so-called) are really smaller in the capacity of their trunks and pelves, and hence less adapted for the duties of motherhood.

The neck carries the head, the legs carry the trunk, and certainly heavy heads and heavy trunks are more safely carried on supports not too long in the perpendicular. This being so, all the data given in our tables of how much you ought to weigh if you are of a given

height require to be revised ; for
any one whose attention has been
called to the subject can readily see
that there are many little people
who are tall, and very many big
people who are short. There are,
of course, a few people—very few,
really—who are both big and tall.
As a rule, very tall people are not
of great constitutional power,
though some tall thin people are
very tough and wiry, and exceedingly vital.

What have height and weight
and their relative merits to do with
gout ? Just this : every little
medico thinks he knows all about
the diet suitable for this ailment
and that, and is so very sure that
a person of a given height should

only weigh so much, and that a big gouty individual may be safely and profitably starved till his height and weight proportion tallies with the table published in his text-books, but which tables are based entirely on false data.

In fine, in judging of the diet suitable to a person, keep in view the amount of work he has to do; and before you determine the proper weight of an individual, do not merely consider his height from crown to sole, but rather have greater regard to the diameters of his trunk.

What first led me, twenty odd years ago, to think more closely of what should be the criterion of a person's weight, was the fact that

a friend of mine, commonly called
little, *i. e.* short, *sat at table higher*
than another friend who was
usually considered a big, *i. e.* tall,
man. And from many observations,
I have long since come to the
conclusion that the big may be
short and the tall small. Also that
the power of an individual is in
proportion, not merely to his hight,
but to *all* his measurements, and
these must be carefully considered
before a true conclusion can be
arrived at.

Hohenheim on the nature of Gout.

Paracelsus' conception of the
true nature of gout *is* true to Nature,
and tallies exactly with my own.

He says (*Tract.* iv., *De origine morb. ex tartaro ;* and in *Erfahrungsheillehre,* p. 95):—"Each organ has the power to separate the huetful from the harmless, and when in this faculty it goes astray, there we get tartarus ;" and thus, for Paracelsus, tartarus is that which ought to have been excreted, but is not, and remains in the body as hurtful material, producing mechanical irritation. Thus stone in the kidneys, bladder, liver, lungs, intestines, under the tongue, or in other regions, is tartarus, and also acidity in the stomach and bowels. Now, put the word *gout* in the place of *tartarus,* and we clearly see that Paracelsus knew as much of the true nature of gout as we of to-day who talk of the uric acid diathesis

6

and the like. Moreover, he knew
how to dissolve stone in the living
body, at which the scholastic wise-
acres have been laughing all my
life, and yet they now howl at those
who question the power of the
much advertised *Piperazine* to do
the same.

Rademacher's Treatment of Gout.

Our author claims that gout
may be caused by a primary disease.
of any given organ or part, or of the
entire organism, and maintains that
in the former case it is curable by
the appropriate organ remedy, while
in the latter case it is curable by
one of the three paracelsic universal
or catholic remedies, *i.e*, nitre, iron,

or copper. So that in this latter
case gout may be of nitric, cupric, or
ferric quality.

Case of Gouty Gastralgia of
Thirteen Years' Duration
Cured by *Urticaurens*.

Not long since a gentleman of
60 years of age, who had lived many
years in a sub-tropical country, came
under my observation for gastralgia
extending right up through the
chest. Although he had lived in
parts where ague is very common,
he is not aware that he has ever
had ague himself. He has many
gouty deposits all over his body,
mostly in the neighbourhood of the
joints. His throat is gouty, and also
his left conjunctiva. There is a

good deal of bronchial catarrh.
The gastralgia yielded quickly and
completely to *Urtica urens,* much
to the amazement of the patient,
who has been under fully a score of
physicians in different parts of the
world for this gastralgia, but in
vain ; and when I first saw him he
was just back from Aix-les-Bains,
which had also done his gastralgia
no good.

The Treatment of The Constitutional Basis of Gout : The Uric Acid Diathesis.

The gouty attack being disposed of, we now come to the real problem, viz., to the cure of that in a given constitution which ends in the deposit of the urate of sodium in the tissues. Th problem is very complex and varied, and it is not easy to explain to the uninitiated that you constitutional anomaly, which we now call the uric acid diathesis, may require very different remedies according to the individual patient. And here it is not a question of the comparative merits of homoeopathy and of allopathy, for allopathy offers us no help, even in theory, for the diathesis. When it is merely a question of the morbid product of the gouty attack, allopathy has a pretty big word to say, either with the *Gichtwasser* or the alkaline treatment, of whose temporary efficacy there can be no doubt, just as there can be no doubt that allopathic remedies open people's bowels; but the alkalies do not cure the gouty constitution any more than do opening medicines cure constipation. To cure constipation, we must have homoeopathy, and so we must correct the gouty diathesis.

The only efficacious plan is to begin by making a diagnosis of the constitutional wrong, and curing that. It may lie in the liver or spleen, or in the kidneys or bowels.* The hapatics often render the very greatest aids : *Chelidonium, Chelone, Carduus, Myrica cerifera, Diplotaxis tenuifolia, Cholesterinum ;* often pancreatics render eminent services, such as *Iris versicolor, Nux vomica, Pulsatilla, Mercurius, Iodine, Jaborandi,*

---

* See Rademacher.

and *Pilocarpine*, used as they may be called for.

Bryonia, too, is often indicated, as also *Sulphur* and *Heparsulphuris*.

We also find, as very frequently indicated, the commoner splenics, such as the already many times mentioned *Urtica urens*, the *Persicaria urens*, the *Rubia tinctoria*, the *Spiritus glandinm quercus*, and the like.

In the renal sphere we may need *Coccus cacti*, *Coccinella*, *Solidago virga aurea*, etc. Going over the notes of some of my cases I find that *Sulphur*, *Thuja*, *Sabina*, *Pulsatilla*, *Bryonia*, *Rhus tox.* *Lycopodium*, and *Antisycotic nosodes* are most commonly to the fore.

But, which of all these ?

In ultimate court of appeal there remains the priceless *Repertory* to lead us to the correct choice of the remedy. With me, personally, the *Repertory* has always been my reserve force, to be called out only in case of need; but, for all that, I feel and know full well that, with my *Repertory* in reserve, I am *never* quite beaten.

The acids in the treatment of gout I have used much and often— of course in repeated doses—*Uric acid* itself (and also *Urea, Urate of sodium,*) *Citric acid, Nitric acid, Hydrochloric acid,* and *Lactic acid.*

Acids are almost universally condemned in the treatment of gout; but, for all that, acids and not alkalies are capable of curing certain cases of gout, only, of course, they must be homoeopathically administered, or you merely add fuel to the flames, and this simple lesson is so hard to learn. Most medical authors, in treating of oxaluria, were against the use of sorrel, rhubarb, and gooseberries, as containing *Oxalic acid.* But these authors might readily observe that although the consumption of a dish of stewed rhubarb is followed by a notable increase in the oxalates, a very notable decrease in the same immediately follows.

Is Fruit Good or Bad For The Gouty ?

I have myself cured gout over and over again with grapes taken in bulk; and several of my patients, who were formerly sorely plagued with gout, have entirely ceased to be troubled so long as they have partaken freely of grapes.

I may say the same of oranges. In fact my standing advice to my gouty friends runs thus :—Eat *plenty* of fresh, ripe, uncooked fruit, and drink *plenty* of fresh cold water. But this advice needs to be somewhat elaborated, for a violent attack of gout may be produced by fruit, particularly where it has been long

eschewed ; and severe gouty head-
aches and bilious attacks may likewise be called forth by partaking
of fresh fruit.

How, then, can we commend
fruit to the gouty ?

It is in this wise : fresh fruits stir
up the gout and often render its
manifestations more active ; but,
at the same time, its tendency is to
diminish gout, and, finally, to get
rid of it, in some cases, altogether.

A *very* little fruit, in a very
gouty individual who is unaccus-
tomed to it, will punish the patient
very severely, as the numberless
stories related by the gouty amply
testify.

"If I eat one gooseberry only, my inside is like a hot cauldron, and all my gouty joints smart fearfully."

"I ate half an apple, and writhed in agony half the night."

And so forth.

All this is quite true, and is indeed within my own professional experience, but at the same time I emphatically state and maintain that fruit is very good for the gouty, for the more fruit they eat the less gout they will (by-and-by) have. Only I will recommend the fruit-eating to be begun with caution, and slowly increased till it becomes not only a harmless but a most beneficent anti-gout habit.

The same remarks apply to *gouty eczema*, which I have often cured; and I am in the habit of telling my patients that I do not consider a case of gouty eczema wholly and radically cured till they can eat fruit freely with impunity. How often do we hear, "Oh, I dare not touch fruit, or I immediately get eczema?" Fruit does *not produce* gout, it stirs it up and drives it out; fruit does *not produce* eczema, it stirs it up and drives it out; and, pray, where is it safest to have gout and eczema? Surely *not* inside.

Do Vegetables and Fruit Conduce to Longevity ?

I am much disposed to answer this question in the affirmative, though my experience and knowledge are not sufficient to supply me with facts and arguments to prove the proposition.

Some years since I knew a gentleman who regarded all fruits and vegetables as *posion*. He died of pure senile decay at 60 years of age. For many years he had eaten neither fruits nor vegetables, but plenty of meat.

A few years previously I knew a West End physician who likewise condemned fruits and vegetables as *rubbish.* He died suddenly about 60 years of age.

And altogether I have long been of opinion, from observation, that those who partake of no vegetables or fruit do not, as a rule, attain to any great age. Oddly enough, I was arguing this question only a few weeks ago with a gentleman of 62 years of age, who had remarked to me that he never ate either fruit or vegetables. Two days thereafter he suddenly expired in a hansom cab while driving across London. His tissues were in a sad state of senile decay.

That the tissues of those who eat neither fruit nor vegetables show grave signs of senility already

at or about middle life is, for me,
almost beyond question ; but
whether the want of the vegetable
causes the decay, or whether the
decay is due to a morbid cause
resulting in a dislike for fruits and
vegetables, as well as in senility, I
am unable to say.

Idiosyncrasy.

In all questions of diet certain
personal peculiarities are to be
respectfully regarded. We do not
know everything. I have lately
been told of a gentleman who gets
severe glossitis from even a spoon-
ful of oaten porridge ; certain
people cannot eat mussels, apples,
strawberries, pork, and so on.
Those idiosyncrasies must be regarded.

On The Influence of Gonorrhœa On The Production of The Gouty Diathesis.

The question of the influence of gonorrhoea upon the constitution has often occupied the minds of thoughtful physicians. At the beginning of this century the *Tripperseuche*, in the German medical thought world, was fairly in the enjoyment of medical citizenship, and it really constitutes the third member in the tripartite pathology of Hahnemann—viz., his sycosis ; and Grauvogl's Hydrogenoid Constitution is another way of putting the same thing. With the advent of the era of Ricord in venereal affections, the *Tripperseuche* was entirely banished, covered with

ridicule. However, it survived in
the homoeopathic school more or
less waningly till a few years ago,
when it came very near death,
except with a certain few of the
Hahnemanninas. Then all at once,
not so long ago, the *Tripperseuche*
was rediscovered by a New York
German physician, who took it
back with him on his return to the
German fatherland, whence it has
spread afresh in thin lines the world
over ; and in France the view that
gonorrhoea is a grave constitutional
disorder is at the present time fash-
ionable. The fact is, Eisenmann's
Tripperseuche will be quite orthodox
again shortly if the present-day
rediscoveries go on much longer.
I have held with Eisenmann,
Hahnemann, Grauvogl, Wolf,

Goullon, these twenty years, and I will just say here that I believe the malady in question has a very decided influence on the organism, being contingently capable of generating a constitutional state which cannot be distinguished from the uric acid diathesis. My conception of the thing is that the gonococcic virus so poisons the organism that acid dypepsia is set up, and then we have what cannot be distinguished from the uric acid diathesis. So often have I seen this state set up in the wake of the gonorrhoeal infection, that I have almost come to the conclusion that the typical gouty attack is a child of gonorrhoea. Thus I explain to myself the curious fact that it is principally men who get

the typical gouty attack. And it
is in this line of thought that I have
met with my greatest success in
the medical eradication of the
uric acid diathesis. But this is a
subject by itself which I may one
day work out; however, in case
I should not do so, let my
advice to the initiated be to this
effect :—Regard the uric acid
diathesis as originating (at least
very frequently) in the *Tripperseuche*, and in its medicinal treatment
stick to the antisycotics, and always
remember its autoison in very high
potency at considerable intervals.
Let it be well understood that I am
here speaking of the uric acid
diathesis, and not of the uric acid
deposits. It is of the very highest
importance always to keep in one's

mind the diathesis separate from
the gouty attack and the gouty
tophi. The homoeopathicity of
the remedy to the diathesis is
mainly historic ; the homoeopathicity of the remedy to the attack is
mainly present and actual. It is
just because these two are considered together that the homoeopathic literature of gout is so poor.
And that others have thought of
the sycotic nature of arthritis may
be inferred from the fact that *Thuja
occidentalis* has been recommended
as an anti-arthritic ; but clearly it
was so recommended for the arthritic
dyspepsia, and not for the arthritic
attack ; and hence we are not
surprised to find that, having used
it in the attacks without benefit,
they have written of *Thuja* as

useless in gout. In the attacks it is indeed useless ; in the arthritic dyspepsia it is a princely remedy.

Case Of Chronic Gout in the Feet and Ankles.

In the spring of 1891 I was requested to go some distance into Surrey to see a lady of 60 years of age who was bedridden for many months from gout in her feet and ankles. It had started, so it was said, from a chill caught while sitting at a railway station waiting for a train. The feet were swelled, very hot, reddish, stiff, and so painful that the patient swooned when I pressed them but gently. There was persistent insomnia and great depression of spirits. After a year's treatment she was discharged quite well, and has since so remained, and with rather unusual activity of limb. The fact is, having been for a time deprived of the use of her feet, and recovered the same only by slow degrees, she set greater value on her power of loco-motion then ever before in her life. She had the following remedies, in the order named—*Urtica urens* θ, *Cypripedium pub.* θ. *Apis mel.* 3^x, *Menyanthes trifoliata* 3^x, *Bellis perennis* θ, and *Viscum album* 1, and after the use of the last named, patient walked from two to four miles a day, with comfort, pleasure, and satisfaction. And the cure holds good to date.

Gouty Insomnia.

A gentleman, 80 years of age, formerly in the army, came under my observation on February 17, 1893, for insomnia, distinctly due to his being full of gout. "I cannot get any sleep without chloral; as soon as 1 lie down at night I get hot, burning, and itchy." His gouty eczema he had got a little under with the aid of sulphur baths. I ordered him *Urtica urens* θ, 10 drops in water, three times a day.

March 3.—"This medicine has done me an immensity of good, but has given me nettle-rash!"

And *apropos* of nettle-rash, everybody knows that the name of the rash is due to the power of the nettle to produce just this kind of rash ; those who question this can readily put into the test of practical scientific experiment by handing a few nettles with gloveless hands. I have very often cured nettle-rash with the nettle-tincture, as so many others have done before me.

It seems to me that if any honest enquirer is really desirous of putting the truth of homoeopathy roughly, yet readily, to the test, he need only handle a few nice nettles with gloveless hands, when he will find that nettles really *do* produce nettle-rash; and then if he will treat a few cases of nettle-rash, occurring as a disease, with some nettle-tea or tincture, he will find that the nettle really does cure the disease nettle-

7

rash ;   . . .   and, if that is not homoeopathy, pray what *is* it ?

Gouty Fistula.

Although fistula is not frequently primarily due to gout, still I have met with some cases of fistula distinctly of a gouty nature.

In the month of January, 1893, a gentleman, 30 odd years of age, sought my advice in regard to a fistula in ano--external and incomplete—that had started with an abscess about a year before. After treating him for some time on the same lines which I commonly follow in the treatment of fistula, I found there was a something present barring progress towards a proper

constitutional cure. And just when
I thought we were at the end of our
task, the fistula suddenly inflamed,
and it was not until patient had
had a course of *Urtica* for a while,
and finally, after taking *Spiritus
glandium quercus* for some six
months with interruptions, that he
reported himself as quite cured.
He had what might very properly
be called fistulitis from indulgence
in drink, and each time it yielded
very speedily to *Quercus*. Patient
himself soon found out which of the
remedies did the good, for on one
occasion, being at a distance, he
telegraphed for this particular medicine. The fact is, the bouts of
acute fistulitis followed immediately
on certain champagne breakfasts
and lobster suppers,

The *Spiritus glandium quercus* has helped me promptly in several other cases of fistula in which the fistulas had become constitutional issues for the excess of alcohol taken into the economy. There are certain cases of fistula that are due almost solely to alcoholism, and these fistulas are simply issues. Woe to the patients if these fistular issues are cured (?) by operation.

The Heart and Kidney Affections Following in the Wake of Gout.

Having gone over some of the main points in the treatment of the gouty attack and the gouty diathesis, we come now to a consideration of

these affections of heart and kidneys that follow in the wake of
gout; and indeed it is here that we
have the most difficult duties to
perform and the most complicated
problems to solve. I mention the
heart and kidney affections as being
of primary and vital importance ;
but in truth there is no single part
of the economy that remains in a
really sound condition, for with
cardiac deterioration there is, *pari
passu,* also a degraded state of the
arteries certainly, and perhaps of
the veins, and in equal step with
this the liver is inadequate, the
digestion is painful and laborious,
the bowels constipated, the throat
may be relaxed and catarrhal, and
attacks of angina. pectoris, gastralgia, and "spasms" are far from

infrequent. The skin, too, is almost sure to show signs of malnutrition, eczema being very common; and vascular naevi, senile warts, and the like are very often met with. It necessarily lies beyond the scope of this volume to discuss the treatmemt for all these ailments, but a short glance at the main medicines will not be out of place.

A very frequently indicated remedy is gold—*Aurum*, either the *Aurum metallicum*, the *Aurum muriaticum*, or the *Aurum muriaticum natronatum*. And this remedy is all the more frequently called for on account of the past histroy of some of the worst cases of post-arthritic heart affections.

Strophanthus—I generally use the first centesimal dilution—helps much, notably where the mishcief lies as between and concerning the liver and the right side of the heart

Where fatty decay is a prominent feature *Phosphorus* does good, but *Vanadium* is here my sheet-anchor —it meets the atheroma of the arteries of brain and liver to a nicety, and thus fills a unique place as being a real remedy of this organic change, and, as an alternate remedy, *Bellis perennis* is a princely medicine.   *Vanadium* 5 and *Bellis* θ month about (with an intercurrent hepatic or two) have in my hands, time and again, restored veritable physical wrecks to health.

Digitaline 2^x (Keith's) ever holds its own as a cardiac tonic. *Convallaria majalis,* too, is a sure friend in the gouty heart, and the same may be affirmed of *Cactus grandifloris.* The liver, pancreas, and spleen lie physically between the heart aud kidneys, and must be concomitantly considered in some cases. The gouty dyspepsia having had its hearing, the kidney troubles proper loom large in the graver cases, and need the very greatest attention, as in them lie the ground causes of so many constitutional upbreakings. Above all things in this regard we must take into account the state of the arteries as leading up to the shedding of the epithelial cells and the exudation of albumen.

Where there is grit and gravel
present, I have had cause to be
satisfied with *Urticus urens* θ and
Coccus cacti θ in alternation at the
beginniug of the treatment, but
their action is not very deep-going.
Where the urine is muddy, pea-
soupy, the ancient *Solidago virga
aurea* θ soothes the kidneys gently
—I had almost said sweetly—5
drops in a tablespoonful of water
is my usual dose.   But *Solidago* is
also a not very deep-going remedy.
Coccinella septempunctata acts very
like it, but goes down a little deeper
and stands midway between it and
Cantharis, which fits the hot con-
gestive quality of nephritis, but the
dose must be infinitesimal.   Where
there is renal bleeding, *Terebinth*
(not lower than the 3ˣ) has classic

claims on our attention. *Phosphoric acid*—about No. 1—is very soothing to the kidneys when the urine is notably phosphatic. In Bright's disease a past grand master in therapeutics has all his work cut out, and he will need all his knowledge, however great, of climate, diet, raiment, and therapeutics. The remedy which, taken by itself, has done most in my hands in chronic Bright's disease is *Mercurius*, about the third trituration. A tincture of cloves, in the same strength, will bring down the quantity of albumen excreted very frequently, and concomitantly there-with there is a rise in patient's feeling of well-being. Considering that cloves cause albuminuria, their use as a condiment should be condemned and forbidden. But the more gentle renal remedies, such as *Solidago*, *Coccinella*, and *Coccus cacti*, are very soothing and helpful in alternation with these deeper-going remedies capable of inducing, and curing, organic change. It is often very helpful in chronic gouty kidney to consider the patient in his or her entirety, and not forget the patients while studying their kidneys. We shall often find that the kidneys are spokesmen for themselves first certainly, but for the liver, heart and arteries, *and skin*, and, indeed, I would affirm of the organ which we call the kidney and of the organism, that the organ speaks for the organism and the organism speaks for the organ, each one "for self and partner.

Gouty Eczema.

This is an affection on which I claim to speak with authority, as I have seen a good deal of it, and know how to cure it. For my general views of the nature of cutaneous affections I refer my readers to my small book, entitled *Diseases of the Skin*.

In general, it will be found that gouty eczema is of a twofold nature, and, not infrequently, of a threefold nature, which can be very prettily demonstrated during one's clinical work, provided the sufferers are patient, which is not always the case, for patience is not commonly an attribute of your gouty person. Your thoroughly gouty individual

may have himself well in hand, and
always stop to dot his i's and cross
his t's and make no use of unscrip-
tural expletives, but he is at best
a pent-up volcano. He may be
very suave and gentle, yielding
and complaisant, but that is from
principle, or training, or pride ; *au-
naturel* he is a wild creature, and
his subject state is the result of
taming. He particularly wants his
gouty eczema cured quickly ; the
nasty thing must be got rid of right
away, and hence he falls a ready
prey to the skin doctors, who know
so little and are so dangerously
shallow that they can confidently
and conscientiously tell you that
the skin affection is a merely local
affair, which lanoline or ichthyol,
with a due proportion of carbolic,

will readily cure. These medicators really believe that a new fat is a medical discovery of the first magnitude, and yet, in very truth, neither ichthyol, nor lanoline, nor vaseline is one whit more of a cure for skin diseases than the good old pig's lard or a tallow candle.

We have had a vaseline era in dermatology, then came the era of lanoline, and at present we are basking in the full glory of the era of ichthyol, and it is all as inane as we can well imagine.

To cure gouty eczema we require patience and perseverence of no ordinary kind, and all the resources of a scientific pharmacology.

Thanks to one Samuel Hahnemann, we *have* a scientific pharmacology, and its data may be found
in Allen's *Encyclopædia of Materia
Medica Pura.*

How long does it take to cure
gouty eczema ?

Speaking for myself, I may say
that I rarely succeed under a year
or a year and a half, and it is
often longer, and sometimes much
longer, but *then* I really cure.

The first principle in the treatment of gouty eczema is negative :
use no external applications whatever, for the affection is not only
constitutional, but it is also mostly
compound and complex in its

nature ; and, I declare most emphatically, that the external treatment of gouty eczema is most dangerous—nay, I would say that it is positively idiotic. Surely, if we have a disease it is better outside than inside, and it, in the end, does not help us to lay the flattering unction to our souls that *our* family blood is faultlessly pure when it is not. "There is no disease in our family," one often hears ; but is it so ? Certain breeds are stronger than others, and given families in their blood-lives are relatively less impure than certain others, but people of absolutely clean, pure blood *I have never known.* Our family taints are printed in our skins in very bold type indeed,—only, happily, not every one can read the record.

Where the gouty eczema has become the cutaneous outlet for the constitution, its uric nature has to be borne in mind, and, in such cases, *Acidum uricum* 6, *Urea* 6, and *Acidum lacitum* 6, render notable service.

Where there is much irritation I have used *Persicaria urens* 6, 12, 30, with much benefit.

Where the whites of the eyes are dirty-looking and lustreless, *Euonymus taropurp.*, *Diplotaxis* θ, and other hapatics are great favourites of mine in gouty eczema.

Where there is a demonstrable sycotic taint, I use all the antisycotics—such as *Thuja*, *Sabina*, *Acid. nit.*, *Cupressus*, *Medorrh.*—

with a free hand, but mostly in
high and higher potencies at infrequent intervals. And every organ
disease must be put right by its
appropriate organ remedies.

Mercurius, Hepar, and *Rhus ven.*
are also frequently indicated. Occasionally, when the wetting ooze
dries up in layers, *Castor equi* has
helped me. When the skin is
brown, or has brown patches, *Sepia,
Iodium,* and *Bacillin* and *Choles-
terin* are friends in need and indeed. The ultimate court of appeal
is the *Materia Medica Pura ;* and
the *Repertory* shows the way to
discover the right remedies. As
a very needful check on aimless
wanderings in this field, however,
we find an accurate knowledge of

the pathology—the morbid biology—of the case in point, and
if to this we add the fundamental
principle, that in scientific therapeutics the cutative range of a
given remedy is fixed by its pathogenetic powers and possibilities, we
are pretty sure to reach the goal.
You cannot, however, hit the target
a mile off with a gun that only
carries fifty yards—no remedy is
therapeutically greater than is the
drug pathogenetically.

INDEX.